"From The Apothecaries Apprentice Journal's Series"

Using the Power of Onions to Treat Respiratory Infections

By Lawrence Pate III

ISBN: 9798644124053

TABLE OF CONTENTS

Introduction

Onions are packed with Vitamin C, and can help boost the immune system and offer protection against bacterial infection and virus. Onions can cure a cold, cough, high fever, sore throat and also boosts immunity.

Please understand, healing through plants is not a one pill, one dose, instant answer to everything. It takes consistency and discipline to stay well. Our bodies get attacked over 8,500 times a day, and in many ways. Usually by things we can't even see. Healing through eating onions seems too easy, but I assure you, it's not. Onions have a profound reaction in our bodies. From re-growing hair to destroying and expelling toxins, and when you add them in herbal healing mixes, the effects are down-right extraordinary.

All of these recipes are best taken with a spoon full of turmeric, and a pinch of black pepper.
Or to be specific:
1 tsp or (3) '00 capsules of turmeric 1/16 tsp of black pepper. If you and yourself really sick. Consume one of these recipes every 3 hours with turmeric and pepper.

For those who already have a virus or know someone who has a virus or for those who have a fever and might be very sick, start reading at Recipe 3

What You Will Need

There are many different stengths of onions.
Green stemmed shallots:
Easiest for kids to eat. Especially when boiled, steamed, or make into a tea (recipes below).
Then there are: leeks, red onions, brown onions, and white onions. I mainly use red and brown as a preference.

Here's your grocery list for the recipes included in this book.
You will need:
Onions- green shallots and brown onion
Fresh garlic cloves
Cayenne pepper powder (90 k H.U. if you can find it)
Raw Honey
Black pepper
Turmeric powder
Chaga mushroom tea bags
Nettle tea bags
  Elderberries
    Fresh ginger

Disclaimer:
Of course by law we cannot guarantee or claim a cure to anything, and that's why we don't claim or guarantee any type of cure for anything. It is always best to check with your doctor and see what's going on inside you first, then attempt to research a treatment.

Recipe #1

(For ages 5 and up)

<u>Tea for Colds</u>

If you feel a cold coming on, you will need:

2 green shallot onions

1 tsp. of turmeric

1/16 tsp. black pepper

Raw Honey

Tea of your choice (I like tangerine tea.)

>Note:

Concerning turmeric, you will need to swallow the powder, not the pills. If all you have is pills, empty them into a measuring spoon to get a full teaspoon. Warning: This will not taste good, but you want the turmeric and pepper to completely cover your whole throat, all the way down.

Directions:

Put 1 tsp of turmeric powder and a pinch (1/16 tsp) of black pepper in your choice of tea or water. Add honey to taste if desired, but no artificial sweeteners.

With the drink, eat 4 inches of raw, uncooked, cleaned, green shallot onions. Take this twice a day.

Recipe #2

(For children, ages 1-5)

Green Shallot Onion Tea
You will need:
(2) - 4 inch pieces of green shallot onion
12 ounces of fresh squeezed orange juice
1/2 inch of fresh ginger

<u>Directions:</u>
Put onions and orange juice in blender. Blend until completely smooth. May add honey to blender to make sweeter if desired, but no artificial sweeteners. Give them at least 2 ounces of this juice every 3 hours.

Recipe #3

Upper Respiratory Infection Specialty Tea (For ages 9 and up)

This is for those who already have a virus or know someone who has a virus or for those who have a fever and might have the virus. If you don't have access to everything on the list just start with onions, warm water, and follow the rest of the directions. Just know everything works better together.

You will need:
1 organic brown onion
 2 tb Elderberries
3 cups of purified water
Raw honey
1 tsp or 1 tea bag Chaga mushroom
(mushroom is optional if allergic to them)
1/16 tsp of black pepper.
1 tsp or (3) '00 capsules of turmeric

*Pick a relaxing tea you like. Here are some suggestions: chamomile, caffeine free peppermint tea, or Lavender honey tea (is my favorite).

Directions:
In a pot, pour water, add chaga tea, elderberries, and relaxing tea of your choice. Bring to a boil, then cut heat off and let steep and cool for 10 -15 mins. Strain and serve. If you don't have relaxing tea, you may: Boil 2 strong cough drops, (preferably Halls with 7.5 mg of

Menthol (listed on the back of package), and stir until dissolved, sweeten to taste.

In a separate cup, mix the turmeric and black pepper well with spoon. (To be clear, don't use pills. Use powder. It will NOT taste the best but you will need the turmeric to cover your throat going down).

Take a brown onion. Cut a slit in the side from top to bottom. Peel the top, dry, layer off and throw it away. Peel off the next juicy layer all the way around, once peeled, seperate into 4 sections, right before you eat the onion, pour the turmeric and pepper in your mouth and quickly drink it down with the warm tea. May take a few swallows.

Then immediately follow the turmeric mix with the 1st section of the onion, repeat again, quickly chase each bite of onion with the warm, well sweetened beverage. Eat 1 to 2 layers twice a day.

It is important to note that raw, brown onions may heat up your mouth. Much like raw garlic or cayenne. This is normal. It is also important to note that if you have a lot of congestion, raw onion acts like a natural expectorant, and may expel the phlegm out of your chest. If your stomach starts to hurt a bit from the onion, that's normal, just pause for an hour letting your stomach digest and continue until the onion is all gone.

Recipe #4

<u>Broccoli and Onion Tea.</u> This one is great for kids who are sick. The tea and honey seems to mask the onion and broccoli taste, but not the smell. It will taste good and smell like the veggies they are.

There are two ways of making this.
<u>You will need:</u>
1 cup of broccoli
1 cup of chopped brown onions
2 cups of water
Honey
<u>Directions:</u>
In a pot, add onions and broccoli, cover with water.
Boil for 15 mins., turn off heat, and let cool to warm, usually about another 10 mins. Strain veggies and set aside. (Can use leftover veggies in a banana, cinnamon and cashew milk shake later). Add organic raw honey to tea, or organic raw sugar only.
*Processed refined sugars of any kind can add inflammation to the body and make a cold worse. (Just changed you life with that one!) Drink your onion broccoli tea with the before mentioned raw onion layers in Recipe #3 as already directed.

A second way to prepare this tea is to add the before mention measurements of broccoli and onion to a liter sized mason jar. Boil 3 cups of puried water, pour water into jar over veggies and let it steep, keep covered for at least 6 hrs. or overnight. Add honey to taste. **This mix will be a bit stronger.

Recipe #5

(For ages 9-99)

<u>Easy Overnight Onion Tea</u>
(This is a bit stronger, for use if you've been sick for over a week)

<u>You will need:</u>
1 brown or white onion
2 nettle tea bags or 1 tbsp of nettle leaf
Honey to taste
Raspberry extract (optional)
<u>Directions:</u>
In a 1 liter mason jar, fill 3/4 full with purified water. Cut up onion and add to jar with nettle tea. Leave in fridge overnight to steep. In the morning, strain out plant matter and sweeten to taste. Can add 5 to 10 drops of raspberry extract for extra favor.

Recipe #6

(For ages 6 months old - 99)

<u>Onions in Honey</u>

One of the simplest cough syrups I know.

<u>Directions:</u>
Cut up a brown onion. Put it in a mason jar. Cover onion with honey and let sit overnight in fridge. Take 1 tsp every 2 to 3 hours until better.

Recipe #7

(For ages 9 -99)

<u>Easy Onion Salad</u>
You will need:
2 cups of spinach
1 brown onion
1 tsp of lemon juice
2 tsp of olive oil
1 clove of garlic
Salt and pepper

<u>Directions:</u>
Cut up onion and garlic. Add as much as you would like.
Mix all ingredients together in a bowl.
Add salt and pepper to taste. Eat and enjoy!

Recipe #8

(For ages 2-99)

<u>Easy Onion Probiotic</u>
Probiotics are good, and healthy bacteria. They are live microorganisms that help prevent and treat illnesses by promoting a healthy immune system and healthy digestion.

<u>You will need:</u>
3 tbsp of sea salt
3 organic red onions
2 quarts of warm purified water
1 liter mason jar with plastic lid
1 (4) oz mason jar with plastic lid
(May need to buy lids separately)

<u>Directions:</u>
Cut onions into slices that can't into mason jar. Fill jar 1/2 full with onions. Add salt. Fill jar 3/4 full with water, and close with top and shake until fully mixed then remove top. All veggies must be completely under salt water by a weight.

<u>To create fermentation weight:</u>
Take smaller 4 oz mason jar, ll with water. Tighten with plastic lid. Flip smaller jar upside down and place in liter jar of onion salt water mix. Press smaller jar, making sure all onions are under water. Make sure that there is at least an inch worth of space at the top of the jar for fermentation to breath. With smaller jar inside larger jar, loosely screw liter jar top down.

-Leave it loose- Do Not tighten-

As the mix ferments, it will bubble and need to breathe. Place the jar in a warm, shady, place, and let sit for 7 to 10 days. Taste every 3 days until you reach a flavor you like. You can keep going with the fermentation until it is as strong as you would like. After about 3 weeks onion smell will go away! Lasts for months. Store in fridge to slow fermentation down once you've reached the taste you

Helpful Tips To Know

*You can cook the onions first to lessen the strength for babies.

*Babies can start eating cooked onions after 6 months.

*Store onions for months in paper bags!

Just dump them into a paper bag and they last for months and months. After some time they will even start regrowing themselves! Keep them out of the fridge, in a cool, dry, shady, place.

With children I find that giving veggies is rarely easy. My kids seemed to like drinking everything from mini cups. Guess it made them feel as big as daddy. But usually, mine would fight to not drink or just throw it up. I got to where I would keep a bowl close by when giving them anything. The first gag and I would ninja that bowl to their bottom lip out of nowhere! I have found that with children, it is more patience and consistency than anything. Eventually kids see that taking plant medicine is not an option. "*You'll stop trying to throw it up before daddy stops trying to make you better*". Sometimes I had to gently remind them, it's either this or the hospital with needles and really sick people.

**This is a handbook of simple, effective, answers and recipes. For many, if it was told to them to do something long and hard, they would gladly do it. But too often, because the answer is simple, many remain sick and in fear because they cannot comprehend and do the simple answer; simple remedies.

Thank You For Your Purchase!

Thank you for your purchase!

This is the 3rd volume in the series of natural remedy recipe books,

"From the Healer's Apprentice Journals."

Please remember that when it comes to organic medicine, not all remedies work for everyone the same. Everyone's health, environment, and living conditions are different. So be safe, careful, and find what works for your situation. Healing is all around us, planted in the Garden God gave us. If you feed your body what it needs to heal itself, it will heal.

Be well, Be Blessed, and Remember....

Plants Are Medicine!

We Welcome Your Feedback!

Feel free to get in touch with us with any feedback or questions.

Email: papabearspantry2019@gmail.com

For Free Recipes Follow me on:

Instagram: www.instagram.com/papabearpantry

Facebook: https://www.facebook.com/Papabear992

Free Fun Facts about Onions:

1) During the American Civil War an onion shortage prompted, General Ulysses S. Grant to send a telegram to the War Department, "I will not move my army without onions." He was immediately shipped three train cars full of onions. In addition to using onions to spice up meals, it was believed the onion had antiseptic properties that could treat wounds.

2) Cultivation of the onion is believed to have begun in Asia around 3500 B.C., However, wild onions grow on nearly every continent. Onions are one of the few vegetables that can easily be stored for the winter. As such, the onion's popularity quickly spread to many cultures.

The onion was worshipped by ancient Egyptians. They believed that   its spherical shape and concentric rings symbolized eternity.

3) Sulfuric compounds in the onion is what makes your eyes tear when cutting onions. The sulfur in onions can also help hair regrow.

-Cut a piece of onion and rub it on your scalp 45 mins before you shower. Then rinse well with your favorite smelling shampoo. After 30 days you will see a difference!

4) To cut down on the crying, chill the onion and cut into

the root end of the onion last. You can also run water while
cutting an onion.

Eating fresh parsley can get rid of "onion breath."

5) World onion production is estimated at approximately 105 billion pounds each year. The average annual onion consumption calculates to approximately 13.67 pounds of onions per person across the world. Libya has the highest consumption of onions with an astounding average per capita consumption of 66.8 pounds. -National Onion Association

The official state vegetable of Georgia is the Vidalia onion.

The official state vegetable of Texas is the Texas Sweet onion.

6) Did you know onion skins contain more antioxidants than the actual onion itself!

Onion skins help lower LDL cholesterol levels!

www.ingramcontent.com/pod-product-compliance
Lightning Source LLC
Chambersburg PA
CBHW031509210526
45463CB00003B/1146